DIABETES GASTROPARESIS DIET COOKBOOK

Quick & Easy Diabetic Delicious Recipes for Gastroparesis to Balanced Blood Sugar, Makes Eating Easier & Digestion Harmony | with 30 Days Meal Plan & Q&A

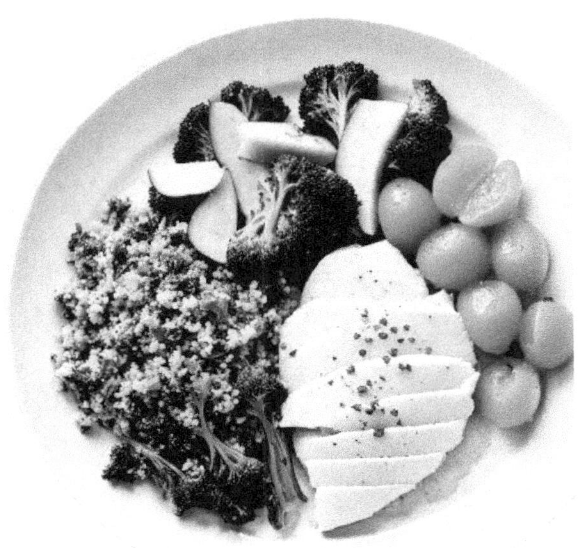

Dr. Margie J. Smith

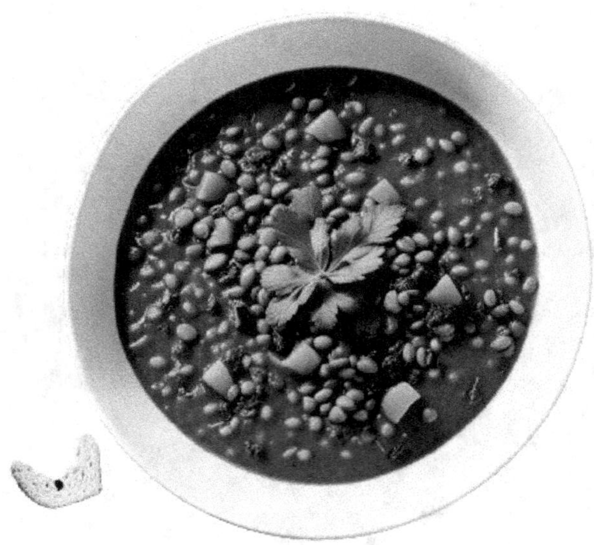

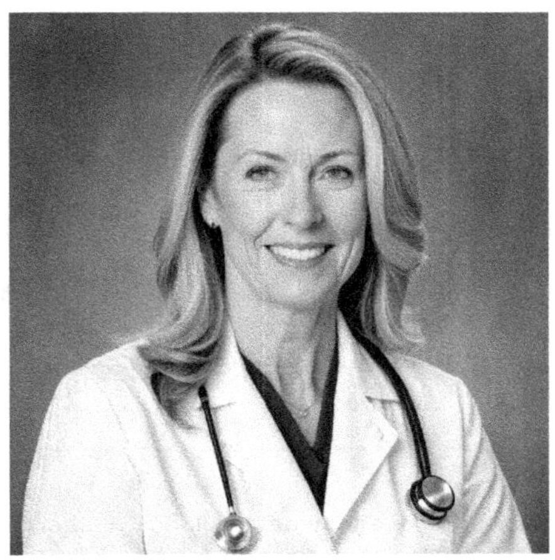

Dr. Margie J. Smith

Hey, I am Dr. Margie J. Smith, just your friendly neighborhood doc, researcher, an' health advocate. You can find me over at Hope Medical Center in the heart of New York City, where I am all about givin' top notch care to everyone who walks through the door. When I am not on duty, you'll catch me chillin' in Greenwich Village, soakin' up the city vibes an' hangin' out with my adorable furball, Whiskers.

My journey into medicine kicked off at Columbia University, where I discovered my love for healin' folks. Then, I headed west for some specialized trainin' at Stanford University. Now, I am all about blendin' the latest research with a big ol' dose of compassion to make sure folks stay healthy an' happy, one patient at a time.

Table of contents

<u>Questions an' Answers</u>

- **What is gastroparesis, an' how does it affect my diet?**

Gastroparesis is a condition that slows down the movement of food through your stomach. This can make digestion difficult an' lead to nausea, vomitin', an' bloatin'. A diabetic gastroparesis diet focuses on easily digestible, low sugar foods to minimize these symptoms an' manage blood sugar levels.

- **Why are there so many recipes with low sugar?**

Both diabetes an' gastroparesis benefit from a low sugar diet. Sugar can be difficult to digest an' can also cause blood sugar spikes in diabetics. This cookbook provides delicious options that won't compromise your health goals.

- **Are there any foods I should completely avoid?**

It's best to discuss specific restrictions with your doctor or registered dietitian. Generally, fatty, greasy, fried foods, processed foods with high sugar content, an' high fiber raw vegetables can be difficult to digest with gastroparesis.

- **Can I still have snacks with this diet?**

Absolutely! This meal plan incorporates healthy an' satisfyin' snacks throughout the day to keep you feelin' full an' prevent blood sugar crashes.

- **What if I don't like the taste of a particular recipe?**

This cookbook offers a variety of options. Feel free to substitute ingredients you enjoy an' explore recipe variations based on your preferences.

- **Are there any specific cookin' techniques I should use?**

Yes, focusin' on gentle cookin' methods like steamin', bakin', poachin', an' simmerin' is ideal for easier digestion. Additionally, you may find it helpful to cut or mash ingredients into smaller pieces.

- **Do I need to drink a lot of water with this diet?**

Stayin' hydrated is crucial for both diabetes an' gastroparesis. Aim to drink plenty of water throughout the day to aid digestion an' manage blood sugar levels.

- **What if I have trouble toleratin' solid foods on some days?**

This meal plan includes options for puréed or soft foods that are easier on the stomach durin' gastroparesis flare ups. Experiment with different textures to find what works best for you on those days.

- **Can I still eat out with this diet?**

Yes, but be mindful of menu choices. Opt for grilled or baked dishes, ask for sauces on the side, an' choose smaller portions.

- **Will I lose weight on this diet?**

Weight loss may occur as a side effect of managin' your conditions. However, the primary focus is on healthy eatin' for improved digestion an' blood sugar control.

- **How often should I be eatin' with this diet?**

Smaller, more frequent meals are generally recommended for both diabetes an' gastroparesis. This helps regulate blood sugar an' reduces the workload on your stomach.

- **Is there a sample meal plan included in the book?**

Yes, the book will provide sample meal plans to give you a startin' point an' demonstrate how to incorporate the recipes into your daily routine.

- **Do I need to see a doctor or dietitian before usin' this cookbook?**

While this book offers valuable information an' recipes, it is not a substitute for professional medical advice. It's crucial to consult your doctor or registered dietitian for a personalized plan that considers your specific needs an' medical history.

- **Where can I find more information about diabetes an' gastroparesis?**

The book may offer resources or suggest reputable organizations for further information. Additionally, you can consult your doctor or search online usin' trusted medical websites.

- **Is there a section on managin' medications alongside this diet?**

This cookbook likely focuses on dietary management. Medication adjustments should be discussed directly with your doctor to ensure optimal control of both diabetes an' gastroparesis.

Introduction

Understandin' Diabetes an' Gastroparesis: A Delicate Balance

For individuals livin' with diabetes, maintainin' a healthy balance is crucial. But what happens when another condition, gastroparesis, enters the equation? This chapter unpacks both conditions an' explores how they can be managed together effectively.

Diabetes 101:

Diabetes mellitus, commonly referred to as diabetes, is a chronic condition affectin' how your body regulates blood sugar (glucose). There are two main types:

- **Type 1 Diabetes**: The body's immune system attacks insulin producin' cells in the pancreas, leadin' to a deficiency of insulin, a hormone needed to transport glucose from the bloodstream into cells for energy.

- **Type 2 Diabetes**: The body either resists insulin's effects or doesn't produce enough insulin.

Regardless of type, uncontrolled diabetes can lead to various complications, includin' nerve damage (neuropathy) an' problems with blood flow.

Gastroparesis in the Spotlight:

Gastroparesis is a digestive disorder that weakens the muscles in the stomach, causin' delayed stomach emptyin'. Food sits in the stomach for an extended period, leadin' to a range of uncomfortable symptoms, includin':

- [ ] Nausea
- [ ] Vomitin'
- [ ] Bloatin'

☐ Early satiety (feelin' full quickly)

☐ Loss of appetite

While the exact cause of gastroparesis is unknown, it can be associated with diabetes related nerve damage or other conditions.

The Two Worlds Collide:

Diabetes an' gastroparesis can create a complex situation. Here's why:

- ❖ **High Blood Sugar**: Uncontrolled blood sugar can worsen gastroparesis by further damagin' the nerves in the stomach.

- ❖ **Dietary Challenges**: Gastroparesis symptoms like nausea an' vomitin' can make it difficult to eat consistently, leadin' to blood sugar fluctuations.

- ❖ **Medication Management**: Both conditions may require medications that can interact or have side effects that complicate the other.

Findin' Harmony:

Despite the challenges, managin' both diabetes an' gastroparesis is possible. Here are some key strategies:

- ❖ **Dietary Adjustments**: Opt for smaller, more frequent meals with easily digestible, low sugar options. This cookbook provides a treasure trove of delicious recipes that fit the bill!

- ❖ **Blood Sugar Monitorin'**: Regularly checkin' blood sugar levels helps identify an' address fluctuations promptly.

- ❖ **Medication Management**: Work with your doctor to ensure medications for both conditions are compatible an' optimized for your needs.

- ❖ **Hydration**: Stayin' hydrated is crucial for both digestion an' blood sugar control.

- ❖ **Communication**: Open communication with your doctor is essential to adjust your management plan as needed.

How This Cookbook Can Help

Jugglin' diabetes an' gastroparesis can feel overwhelmin', especially when it comes to meal plannin'. This cookbook is your partner in navigatin' this delicate balance, offerin' delicious an' practical solutions to help you feel your best.

Here's how this book empowers you:

- ❖ **Variety is Key**: We offer a diverse selection of recipes for breakfast, lunch, dinner, an' snacks, ensurin' you don't get stuck in a rut. From savory frittatas to protein smoothies, explore options that cater to different tastes an' textures.

- ❖ **Low Sugar Focus**: Managin' diabetes is a priority. Every recipe prioritizes low sugar ingredients an' sugar substitutes, allowin' you to enjoy flavorful meals without compromisin' blood sugar control.

- ❖ **Digestive Ease**: Understandin' the limitations of gastroparesis, this cookbook features recipes that are easily digestible. Gentle cookin' methods an' options for puréed or soft foods make mealtimes less stressful on your stomach.

- ❖ **Meal Plannin' Made Simple**: We provide several sample meal plans to kickstart your journey. These plans showcase how to incorporate the recipes into your daily routine, considerin' portion sizes an' meal frequency. Feel free to customize them based on your preferences an' doctor's recommendations.

- ❖ **Beyond Recipes**: This book goes beyond simply providin' recipes. We offer valuable information on managin' both diabetes an' gastroparesis, includin' dietary tips, hydration strategies, an' the importance of communication with your healthcare team.

Imagine this:

1. Startin' your day with a protein smoothie packed with essential nutrients, all while keepin' your blood sugar in check.

2. Enjoyin' a satisfyin' lunch of chicken lettuce wraps with a flavorful peanut sauce, knowin' it is gentle on your stomach.

3. Endin' the day with a delicious baked salmon with roasted vegetables, a complete an' balanced meal that won't cause discomfort.

Chapter 1: Livin' with Diabetes an' Gastroparesis

The Importance of Diet Management

Diet management plays a central role in effectively managin' both diabetes an' gastroparesis. It's a powerful tool that can help you:

For Diabetes:

- **Maintain Healthy Blood Sugar Levels**: By prioritizin' low sugar, balanced meals, you provide your body with a steady stream of energy without causin' blood sugar spikes. This reduces the risk of long term complications associated with uncontrolled diabetes.

- **Promote Weight Management**: Maintainin' a healthy weight can significantly benefit diabetes control. This cookbook offers delicious, yet portion controlled recipes to support a healthy weight range as recommended by your doctor.

- **Reduce Risk of Other Chronic Conditions**: A healthy diet rich in fruits, vegetables, an' whole grains can help lower your risk of heart disease, high blood pressure, an' certain types of cancer   all potential complications of uncontrolled diabetes.

For Gastroparesis:

- **Minimize Symptoms**: Choosin' easily digestible foods an' smaller, more frequent meals reduces the workload on your stomach, potentially leadin' to fewer episodes of nausea, vomitin', an' bloatin'.

- **Maintain Proper Nutrition**: Gastroparesis can make it difficult to get the nutrients your body needs. This book provides recipes packed with essential vitamins an' minerals, ensurin' you stay nourished despite the challenges.

- **Improve Overall Well being**: By managin' gastroparesis symptoms through diet, you'll likely experience increased energy, improved mood, an' a better quality of life.

The Synergistic Effect:

- The beauty lies in the synergy between these benefits. By managin' diabetes through diet, you're also creatin' a foundation for better digestion in gastroparesis. Conversely, choosin' gastroparesis friendly foods often aligns with healthy diabetic choices. This cookbook capitalizes on this connection, offerin' recipes that address both conditions simultaneously.

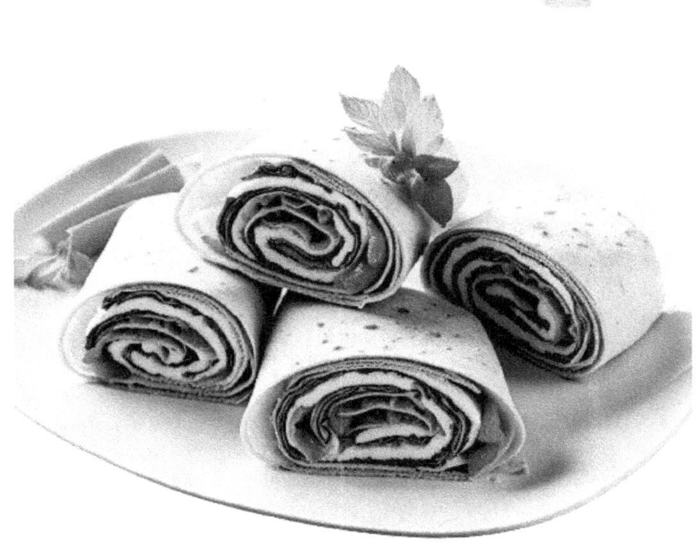

Nutritional Considerations

Managin' both diabetes an' gastroparesis requires a delicate balance between blood sugar control an' promotin' healthy digestion. Here are a few minor dietary considerations to remember:

Carbohydrates:

- **Focus on Complex Carbs**: Choose whole grains like brown rice, quinoa, an' whole wheat bread over refined carbohydrates like white bread, pasta, an' sugary cereals. Complex carbs provide sustained energy without causin' blood sugar spikes.

- **Portion Control is Key**: Even healthy carbs can impact blood sugar. Be mindful of portion sizes an' work with your doctor or dietitian to determine the appropriate carb intake for your needs.

Protein:

- **Prioritize Lean Protein Sources**: Include protein in every meal to promote satiety, support blood sugar control, an' aid in healin' an' repair. Opt for lean protein sources like grilled chicken, fish, turkey, beans, an' lentils.

Fats:

- **Healthy Fats are Your Friend**: Healthy fats like those found in avocados, nuts, seeds, an' olive oil can help with satiety an' nutrient absorption. However, limit unhealthy fats like saturated an' trans fats found in fried foods an' processed meats.

Fiber:

- **Balance is Necessary**: Fiber is crucial for gut health, but it can also slow down digestion, which can be problematic with gastroparesis. Choose soluble fiber sources like fruits (berries are a good option) an' vegetables over insoluble fiber found in whole grains an' nuts. You may need to discuss modifyin' your fiber intake with your doctor or dietitian.

Sugar:

- **Limit Added Sugars:** Added sugars significantly impact blood sugar levels an' offer minimal nutritional value. This cookbook emphasizes recipes with minimal to no added sugar, utilizin' natural sweeteners like stevia or monk fruit extract when necessary.

Fluids:

- **Hydration is Essential**: Stayin' hydrated is crucial for both diabetes an' gastroparesis. Aim to drink plenty of water throughout the day to aid digestion, prevent constipation, an' support overall health.

Vitamins an' Minerals:

- **Nutrient Dense Choices**: Gastroparesis can make it difficult to absorb all the nutrients your body needs. Choose nutrient dense foods like fruits, vegetables, an' lean protein sources to ensure you're gettin' essential vitamins an' minerals.

Additional Considerations:

- **Smaller, More Frequent Meals**: Eatin' smaller meals an' snacks throughout the day is often easier on the stomach than large, infrequent meals. This helps regulate blood sugar an' reduces the workload on your digestive system.

- **Food Consistency**: Experiment with food consistency to find what works best for you. Some may find puréed or soft foods easier to tolerate durin' gastroparesis flare ups.

- **Cookin' Methods**: Gentle cookin' methods like steamin', bakin', poachin', an' simmerin' are ideal for easier digestion. You may also find it helpful to cut or mash ingredients into smaller pieces.

Chapter 2: Low Sugar Recipe Fundamentals

Cookin' Techniques for Easier Digestion

Livin' with both diabetes an' gastroparesis can make mealtimes a challenge. However, focusin' on gentle cookin' methods an' specific food preparation techniques can significantly improve your digestion an' overall experience. This chapter explores some helpful strategies to transform your kitchen into an ally for managin' both conditions.

Gentle Cookin' Methods:

- ★ **Steamin'**: This method uses steam to cook food, preservin' nutrients an' resultin' in a soft, easily digestible texture. Steam vegetables, fish, an' even dumplings for a healthy an' gentle approach.

- ★ **Bakin'**: Bakin' is a versatile technique that allows you to cook a variety of foods without added fats or oils. Roasted vegetables, baked chicken or fish, an' even sweet potato fries are all delicious options that are gentle on the stomach.

- ★ **Poachin'**: Poachin' involves simmerin' food in a flavorful liquid like broth or water. This method results in moist, tender protein sources like chicken, fish, an' eggs, perfect for those with gastroparesis.

- ★ **Simmerin'**: Similar to poachin', simmerin' involves cookin' food in a liquid at a low temperature for an extended period. This allows for tougher cuts of meat to become tender an' flavorful, while remainin' easily digestible.

Food Preparation Techniques:

- ★ **Cuttin' an' Choppin'**: Reduce the size of your food by choppin', mincin', or shreddin' vegetables, fruits, an' even meats. This increases the surface area, allowin' digestive enzymes to work more efficiently.

- ★ **Puréeing**: For days when your digestion feels particularly challenged, consider puréing cooked vegetables, soups, or even cooked meats. This creates a smooth consistency that's effortless to digest.

- ★ **Mashed or Riced**: Similar to puréeing, mashin' vegetables like potatoes or cauliflower creates a softer texture that's easier on the stomach. Riced cauliflower can be a great substitute for grains.

- ★ **Marinatin'**: Marinatin' meats can help tenderize them before cookin', makin' them easier to digest. Use low sugar marinades or create your own with herbs, spices, an' sugar substitutes.

Additional Tips:

- ★ **Low Fat Cookin'**: Limit added fats an' oils when cookin', as they can slow down digestion. Opt for cookin' methods like steamin', bakin', an' poachin' that require minimal added fat.

- ★ **Seasonin' an' Flavor Boosters**: Don't be afraid to experiment with herbs, spices, an' sugar free flavorings. These can add depth an' complexity to your dishes without impactin' blood sugar levels.

- ★ **Smaller Meals, More Frequently**: Opt for smaller, more frequent meals throughout the day to reduce the workload on your stomach. This can also help regulate blood sugar levels.

- ★ **Listen to Your Body**: Experiment with different techniques an' food consistencies to find what works best for you. Some days you may tolerate more solid foods, while others may require softer options.

Tips for Smart Swaps an' Substitutions

Livin' with diabetes an' gastroparesis requires creativity in the kitchen. This chapter empowers you to become a substitution superhero, enablin' you to enjoy delicious meals that fit your dietary needs.

Masterin' Sugar Substitutions:

- **Artificial Sweeteners**: Explore sugar substitutes like stevia, erythritol, or monk fruit extract. Remember, moderation is key, as some artificial sweeteners can cause digestive issues in high doses.

- **Natural Sweeteners**: Utilize natural sweetness from fruits like berries or applesauce. You can also use pureed dates or bananas for a touch of sweetness an' added moisture in bakin'.

Swappin' Carbohydrates:

- **Refined Grains vs. Whole Grains**: Swap out refined carbohydrates like white bread, pasta, an' rice for whole wheat options or alternatives like quinoa, brown rice, or lentil pasta. These provide sustained energy an' essential fiber without the blood sugar spike.

- **Starchy Vegetables**: Be mindful of portions for starchy vegetables like potatoes an' corn, as they can impact blood sugar levels. Explore lower glycemic options like zucchini, spaghetti squash, or cauliflower rice.

Protein Powerhouses:

- **Lean Protein Sources**: Prioritize lean protein sources like grilled chicken, fish, or turkey. You can also explore plant based protein options like beans, lentils, an' tofu.

Healthy Fat Alternatives:

❖ **Healthy Fat Sources**: Include healthy fats from sources like avocados, nuts, seeds, an' olive oil. Limit unhealthy fats like saturated an' trans fats found in fried foods an' processed meats.

Gastroparesis Friendly Tweaks:

❖ **Reducin' Fiber**: If high fiber foods irritate your stomach, opt for cooked or canned vegetables over raw options. You can also remove the skins of fruits an' vegetables to reduce fiber content.

❖ **Liquids over Solids**: On days when your digestion feels compromised, consider smoothies made with low sugar yogurt, protein powder, an' berries. Soups are another excellent option, an' this book offers puréed options for those times.

General Recipe Swaps:

• **Creamy Sauces**: For a lighter alternative to creamy sauces, use low fat Greek yogurt thinned with a little broth or use silken tofu for a thicker consistency.

• **Thickened Soups**: Instead of heavy cream to thicken soups, use mashed cauliflower, xanthan gum, or a cornstarch slurry.

Stockin' Your Pantry for Diabetic Gastroparesis Meals

Conquerin' diabetes an' gastroparesis starts in your pantry. Here's your roadmap to creatin' a well stocked haven filled with ingredients that support both conditions, makin' meal prep a breeze.

Pantry Staples for Diabetes Management:

- ❖ **Low Glycemic Index (GI) Grains**: Focus on whole grains like brown rice, quinoa, whole wheat pasta, an' barley. These provide sustained energy without blood sugar spikes. Consider options like rolled oats for smoothies or overnight oats.

- ❖ **Sugar Substitutes**: Stock sugar substitutes like stevia, erythritol, or monk fruit extract for sweetenin'. Remember, moderation is key!

- ❖ **Dried Fruits an' Nuts**: Keep a selection of unsweetened dried fruits (cranberries, blueberries) an' nuts (almonds, walnuts) for healthy snacks or additions to meals. Opt for unsalted or dry roasted varieties for better sodium control.

- ❖ **Canned Beans an' Lentils**: These are fantastic sources of protein an' fiber, perfect for incorporatin' into soups, salads, or creatin' vegetarian main courses.

- ❖ **Canned Low Sodium Vegetables**: Stock up on a variety of canned vegetables like diced tomatoes, green beans, an' corn. Opt for low sodium options to manage blood pressure.

- ❖ **Healthy Cookin' Oils:** Have a heart healthy oil like olive oil on hand for occasional use in cookin'.

Pantry Essentials for Gastroparesis Friendly Meals:

- ❖ **Low Fiber Vegetables:** Choose softer vegetables like zucchini, yellow squash, carrots (cooked), an' green beans for easier digestion. Frozen options can be a time saver.

- ❖ **Canned or Pouched Tuna an' Salmon**: Canned lean protein sources like tuna an' salmon are excellent options for quick meals or protein additions.

- ❖ **Low Fat Yogurt**: Unsweetened or minimally sweetened yogurt provides protein an' calcium, an' can be used in smoothies or enjoyed with berries as a snack.

- ❖ **Unsweetened Applesauce**: Applesauce is a versatile ingredient, offerin' natural sweetness for bakin' or as a standalone snack.

- ❖ **Smoothie Boosters**: Keep frozen fruits (berries, mango) an' unsweetened nut butter on hand for whippin' up quick an' nutritious smoothies.

- ❖ **Clear Broths**: Low sodium chicken or vegetable broth are essential for creatin' flavorful soups an' can be used to thin sauces for a lighter consistency.

- ❖ **Low FODMAP Options (Optional):** If you suspect FODMAPs (Fermentable Oligosaccharides, Disaccharides, Monosaccharides, an' Polyols) may be triggerin' gastroparesis symptoms, consider low FODMAP alternatives like lactose free yogurt an' gluten free grains (consult your doctor for guidance).

Beyond the Basics:

- ❖ **Spices an' Herbs**: Spices an' herbs add depth of flavor without impactin' blood sugar or digestion. Explore options like gin'er, garlic powder, cinnamon, an' dried basil.

- ❖ **Sugar Free Flavorings**: Consider sugar free extracts like vanilla, almond, or lemon to add a touch of sweetness to yogurt or smoothies.

- ❖ **Non Starchy Thickeners**: Stock up on thickeners like xanthan gum or glucomannan powder for creatin' thicker soups or sauces without relyin' on heavy cream.

RECIPES

Breakfast

Scrambled Eggs with Spinach an' Feta Cheese

Preparation Time: 15 minutes

Ingredients:

- ☐ Eggs
- ☐ Spinach
- ☐ Feta cheese
- ☐ Salt
- ☐ Pepper

Directions:

1. Raise a nonstick skillet to a moderate temperature.
2. Whisk eggs in a bowl an' season with salt an' pepper.
3. Add spinach to the skillet an' cook until wilted.
4. Pour in the eggs an' scramble until almost set.
5. Crumble feta cheese over the eggs an' continue cookin' until eggs are fully set.

Nutrition Info per Servin' (approximately):

- Calories: 250
- Protein: 18g
- Fat: 17g
- Carbohydrates: 5g

Storage an' Freezin':

- Best enjoyed fresh.

Why This Recipe is So Good:

- It's a flavorful an' protein rich breakfast option with the creamy goodness of feta cheese an' the nutritional benefits of spinach.

Protein Smoothie with Berries an' Unsweetened Almond Milk

Preparation Time: 5 minutes

Ingredients:

- ☐ Berries (e.g., strawberries, blueberries)
- ☐ Unsweetened almond milk
- ☐ Protein powder

Directions:

1. Blend berries, almond milk, an' protein powder until smooth.
2. If necessary, adjust consistency by adding more almond milk.
3. Serve immediately.

Nutrition Info per Servin' (approximately):

- Calories: 200
- Protein: 25g
- Fat: 3g
- Carbohydrates: 15g

Storage an' Freezin':

- Best enjoyed fresh.

Why This Recipe is So Good:

- It's a quick an' convenient way to get a protein packed breakfast with the natural sweetness of berries an' the creamy texture of almond milk.

Chia Seed Puddin' with Nut Butter an' Sliced Strawberries

Preparation Time: 5 minutes (plus chillin' time)

Ingredients:

- ☐ Chia seeds
- ☐ Nut butter (e.g., almond butter, peanut butter)
- ☐ Strawberries

Directions:

1. Mix chia seeds with water or milk in a jar or bowl.
2. Stir well an' refrigerate for at least 2 hours or overnight.
3. Serve chilled, topped with a dollop of nut butter an' sliced strawberries.

Nutrition Info per Servin' (approximately):

- Calories: 280
- Protein: 8g
- Fat: 15g
- Carbohydrates: 25g

Storage an' Freezin':

- Chia puddin' can be stored in the refrigerator for up to 3 days.

Why This Recipe is So Good:

- It's a nutritious an' satisfyin' breakfast option loaded with fiber, healthy fats from nut butter, an' the freshness of sliced strawberries.

Baked Oatmeal with Apples an' Cinnamon (use sugar substitutes like stevia)

Preparation Time: 30 minutes

Ingredients:

- ☐ Oats
- ☐ Apples
- ☐ Cinnamon
- ☐ Stevia or other sugar substitutes

Directions:

1. Preheat oven to 350°F (175°C) an' grease a bakin' dish.
2. Mix oats, diced apples, cinnamon, an' stevia in a bowl.
3. Spread mixture into the bakin' dish an' bake for 25 30 minutes, or until golden brown an' set.
4. Serve warm.

Nutrition Info per Servin' (approximately):

- Calories: 220
- Protein: 5g
- Fat: 3g
- Carbohydrates: 45g

Storage an' Freezin':

- Leftovers can be refrigerated an' reheated.

Why This Recipe is So Good:

- It's a comfortin' an' low sugar breakfast option with the natural sweetness of apples an' the warmth of cinnamon.

Savory Frittata with Vegetables an' Goat Cheese

Preparation Time: 25 minutes

Ingredients:

- ☐ Eggs
- ☐ Vegetables (e.g., bell peppers, onions, spinach)
- ☐ Goat cheese

Directions:

1. Preheat oven to 350°F (175°C).
2. Whisk eggs in a bowl an' season with salt an' pepper.
3. Sauté vegetables in an oven safe skillet until tender.
4. Pour eggs over the vegetables an' cook for 3 4 minutes.
5. Crumble goat cheese over the top an' transfer the skillet to the oven.
6. Bake for 10 12 minutes, or until the frittata is set an' cheese is melted.

Nutrition Info per Servin' (approximately):

- Calories: 280
- Protein: 18g
- Fat: 20g
- Carbohydrates: 8g

Storage an' Freezin':

- Frittata can be refrigerated an' reheated.

Why This Recipe is So Good:

- It's a satisfyin' an' protein rich breakfast option with the creamy tanginess of goat cheese an' the freshness of mixed vegetables.

Greek Yogurt with Chopped Nuts an' a sprinkle of berries

Preparation Time: 5 minutes

Ingredients:

- Greek yogurt
- Nuts (e.g., almonds, walnuts)
- Berries (e.g., raspberries, blueberries)

Directions:

1. Spoon Greek yogurt into a bowl.
2. Top with chopped nuts an' a sprinkle of berries.
3. Serve immediately.

Nutrition Info per Servin' (approximately):

- Calories: 220
- Protein: 20g
- Fat: 10g
- Carbohydrates: 15g

Storage an' Freezin':

- Best enjoyed fresh.

Why This Recipe is So Good:

- It's a creamy an' protein packed breakfast option with the crunchiness of nuts an' the burst of flavor from fresh berries.

Cottage Cheese Pancakes with a dollop of sugar free syrup

Preparation Time: 20 minutes

Ingredients:

- ☐ Cottage cheese
- ☐ Eggs
- ☐ Almond flour or oat flour
- ☐ Bakin' powder
- ☐ Sugar free syrup

Directions:

1. Blend cottage cheese, eggs, flour, an' bakin' powder in a blender until smooth.
2. Heat a non stick skillet over medium heat an' pour batter to form pancakes.
3. Cook until bubbles form on the surface, then flip an' cook until golden brown on both sides.
4. Serve with a dollop of sugar free syrup.

Nutrition Info per Servin' (approximately):

- Calories: 200
- Protein: 15g
- Fat: 10g
- Carbohydrates: 10g

Storage an' Freezin':

- Leftover pancakes can be refrigerated or frozen.

Why This Recipe is So Good:

- It's a low carb an' high protein breakfast option with the creaminess of cottage cheese an' the sweetness of sugar free syrup.

Whole Wheat Toast with Avocado an' a sprinkle of Everythin' But the Bagel Seasonin'

Preparation Time: 5 minutes

Ingredients:

- [ ] Whole wheat bread
- [ ] Avocado
- [ ] Everythin' But the Bagel Seasonin'

Directions:

1. Toast whole wheat bread until golden brown.
2. Mash avocado onto the toast.
3. Sprinkle with Everythin' But the Bagel Seasonin'.
4. Serve immediately.

Nutrition Info per Servin' (approximately):

- Calories: 180
- Protein: 5g
- Fat: 10g
- Carbohydrates: 20g

Storage an' Freezin':

- Best enjoyed fresh.

Why This Recipe is So Good:

- It's a simple an' nutritious breakfast option with the creaminess of avocado an' the savory flavor of Everythin' But the Bagel Seasonin'.

Poached Eggs on a bed of wilted greens

Preparation Time: 10 minutes

Ingredients:

- ☐ Eggs
- ☐ Greens (e.g., spinach, kale)

Directions:

1. Fill a skillet with water an' brin' to a gentle simmer.
2. Crack eggs into separate cups.
3. Carefully slide eggs into the simmerin' water an' poach for 3 4 minutes, or until whites are set but yolks are still runny.
4. Meanwhile, sauté greens in a separate skillet until wilted.
5. Serve poached eggs on a bed of wilted greens.

Nutrition Info per Servin' (approximately):

- Calories: 150
- Protein: 10g
- Fat: 10g
- Carbohydrates: 5g

Storage an' Freezin':

- Best enjoyed fresh.

Why This Recipe is So Good:

- It's a simple an' protein rich breakfast option with the creaminess of poached eggs an' the freshness of wilted greens.

Breakfast Sausage Links with Scrambled Egg Whites

Preparation Time: 15 minutes

Ingredients:

- ☐ Breakfast sausage links
- ☐ Egg whites

Directions:

1. Cook breakfast sausage links accordin' to package instructions.
2. In a separate skillet, scramble egg whites until cooked through.
3. Serve sausage links with scrambled egg whites.

Nutrition Info per Servin' (approximately):

- Calories: 220
- Protein: 20g
- Fat: 15g
- Carbohydrates: 2g

Storage an' Freezin':

- Best enjoyed fresh.

Why This Recipe is So Good:

- It's a protein packed breakfast option with the savory flavor of sausage links an' the lightness of scrambled egg whites.

Lunch

Chicken or Turkey Lettuce Wraps with Chopped Vegetables an' a Low Sugar Peanut Sauce

Preparation Time: 15 minutes

Ingredients:

- ☐ Ground chicken or turkey
- ☐ Lettuce leaves
- ☐ Chopped vegetables (e.g., bell peppers, carrots, cucumber)
- ☐ Low sugar peanut sauce

Directions:

1. Cook ground chicken or turkey in a skillet until fully cooked.
2. Wash an' prepare lettuce leaves as wraps.
3. Fill lettuce leaves with cooked meat an' chopped vegetables.
4. Drizzle with low sugar peanut sauce.

Nutrition Info per Servin' (approximately):

- Calories: 250
- Protein: 20g
- Fat: 10g
- Carbohydrates: 15g

Storage an' Freezin':

- Best enjoyed fresh.

Why This Recipe is So Good:
- These lettuce wraps offer a satisfyin' combination of protein an' crunchy vegetables, complemented by a flavorful low sugar peanut sauce.

Lentil Soup with Whole Wheat Bread for Dippin'

Preparation Time: 30 minutes

Ingredients:

- [ ] Lentils
- [ ] Vegetables (e.g., carrots, celery, onions)
- [ ] Vegetable broth
- [ ] Whole wheat bread

Directions:

1. Rinse lentils an' combine with chopped vegetables an' vegetable broth in a pot.
2. Brin' to a boil, then reduce heat an' simmer until lentils are tender.
3. Serve hot with whole wheat bread for dippin'.

Nutrition Info per Servin' (approximately):

- Calories: 200
- Protein: 12g
- Fat: 2g
- Carbohydrates: 35g

Storage an' Freezin':

- You may refrigerate leftover soup for up to three days.

Why This Recipe is So Good:

- Lentil soup is a hearty an' nutritious meal, packed with fiber an' protein, perfect for dippin' with whole wheat bread.

Tuna Salad on a Bed of Romaine Lettuce with Chopped Celery an' Red Onion

Preparation Time: 10 minutes

Ingredients:

- ☐ Canned tuna
- ☐ Romaine lettuce
- ☐ Chopped celery
- ☐ Red onion
- ☐ Dressin' of choice (e.g., vinaigrette)

Directions:

1. Drain canned tuna an' flake into a bowl.
2. Arrange romaine lettuce leaves on a plate.
3. Top lettuce with tuna, chopped celery, an' red onion.
4. Drizzle with dressin' of choice.

Nutrition Info per Servin' (approximately):

- Calories: 180
- Protein: 20g
- Fat: 5g
- Carbohydrates: 10g

Storage an' Freezin':

- Best enjoyed fresh.

Why This Recipe is So Good:

- This tuna salad is a light an' refreshin' option, rich in protein an' fiber, with added crunch from celery an' onion.

Grilled poultry or fish paired with roasted vegetables

Preparation Time: 30 minutes

Ingredients:

- ☐ Chicken breasts or fish fillets
- ☐ Assorted vegetables (e.g., bell peppers, zucchini, cherry tomatoes)
- ☐ Olive oil
- ☐ Salt
- ☐ Pepper

Directions:

1. Preheat grill or oven to medium high heat.
2. Season chicken or fish with salt, pepper, an' olive oil.
3. Grill or bake until cooked through.
4. Meanwhile, toss vegetables with olive oil, salt, an' pepper.
5. Roast vegetables in the oven until tender.

Nutrition Info per Servin' (approximately):

- Calories: 300 (chicken) / 250 (fish)
- Protein: 25g (chicken) / 20g (fish)
- Fat: 10g (chicken) / 8g (fish)
- Carbohydrates: 20g

Storage an' Freezin':

- Best enjoyed fresh.

Why This Recipe is So Good:

- Grilled chicken or fish paired with roasted vegetables is a simple an' wholesome meal, providin' lean protein an' a variety of nutrients from the colorful veggies.

Turkey an' Vegetable Chili (Use No Sugar Added Diced Tomatoes)

Preparation Time: 45 minutes

Ingredients:

- [ ] Ground turkey
- [ ] Assorted vegetables (e.g., bell peppers, onions, tomatoes)
- [ ] No sugar added diced tomatoes
- [ ] Beans (e.g., kidney beans, black beans)
- [ ] Chili powder
- [ ] Cumin
- [ ] Salt
- [ ] Pepper

Directions:

1. In a large pot, cook ground turkey until browned.
2. Add chopped vegetables an' cook until softened.
3. Stir in diced tomatoes, beans, chili powder, cumin, salt, an' pepper.
4. Simmer for 30 minutes, stirrin' occasionally.

Nutrition Info per Servin' (approximately):

- Calories: 280
- Protein: 25g
- Fat: 8g
- Carbohydrates: 30g

Storage an' Freezin':

- Chili can be stored in the refrigerator for up to 3 days or frozen for longer storage.

Why This Recipe is So Good:
- This hearty turkey an' vegetable chili is packed with protein, fiber, an' essential nutrients, makin' it a satisfyin' an' nourishin' meal option.

Leftover Stir Fry from Dinner (Ensure Low Sugar Ingredients)

Preparation Time: 10 minutes

Ingredients:

- ☐ Leftover stir fry (with low sugar sauce)

Directions:

1. Reheat leftover stir fry in a skillet or microwave until heated through.
2. Serve hot.

Nutrition Info per Servin' (approximately):

- ☐ Nutrition varies based on ingredients used in the stir fry.

Storage an' Freezin':

- Best enjoyed fresh.

Why This Recipe is So Good:

- Utilizin' leftovers reduces food waste an' provides a quick an' convenient meal option, ensurin' you're still enjoyin' a balanced an' healthy dish.

Salmon with a Lemon Dill Sauce an' Steamed Asparagus

Preparation Time: 20 minutes

Ingredients:

- ☐ Salmon fillets
- ☐ Lemon
- ☐ Fresh dill
- ☐ Olive oil
- ☐ Salt
- ☐ Pepper
- ☐ Asparagus

Directions:

1. Preheat oven to 375°F (190°C).
2. Season salmon fillets with salt, pepper, an' a squeeze of lemon juice.
3. Place salmon on a bakin' sheet lined with parchment paper an' bake for 12 15 minutes or until cooked through.
4. Meanwhile, steam asparagus until tender.
5. Prepare lemon dill sauce by mixin' fresh dill, lemon zest, lemon juice, olive oil, salt, an' pepper.
6. Serve salmon topped with lemon dill sauce alongside steamed asparagus.

Nutrition Info per Servin' (approximately):

- Calories: 300
- Protein: 25g
- Fat: 15g
- Carbohydrates: 10g

Storage an' Freezin':

- Best enjoyed fresh.

- This salmon dish is not only delicious but also rich in omega 3 fatty acids an' packed with flavor from the lemon dill sauce.

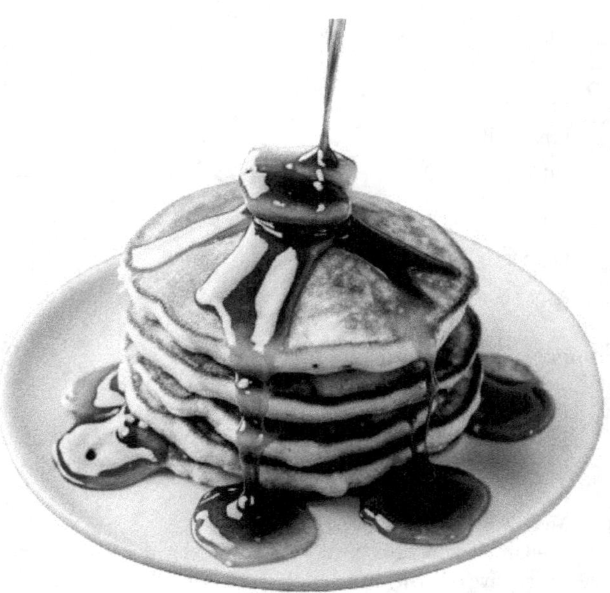

Cold Sesame Noodles with Shredded Chicken an' Vegetables (Use Low Sugar Sesame Sauce)

Preparation Time: 20 minutes

Ingredients:

- [ ] Whole wheat noodles or soba noodles
- [ ] Shredded chicken breast
- [ ] Assorted vegetables (e.g., bell peppers, carrots, cucumber)
- [ ] Low sugar sesame sauce

Directions:

1. Cook noodles accordin' to package instructions, then rinse under cold water an' drain.
2. Toss noodles with shredded chicken an' chopped vegetables.
3. Drizzle with low sugar sesame sauce an' toss to combine.
4. Serve chilled.

Nutrition Info per Servin' (approximately):

- Calories: 320
- Protein: 25g
- Fat: 10g
- Carbohydrates: 30g

Storage an' Freezin':

- Best enjoyed fresh.

Why This Recipe is So Good:

- Cold sesame noodles are a refreshin' dish, providin' a balanced combination of carbs, protein, an' veggies, enhanced by the savory flavors of the low sugar sesame sauce.

Black Bean Burgers on Whole Wheat Buns with a Side Salad

Preparation Time: 30 minutes

Ingredients:

- [ ] Black beans (canned or cooked)
- [ ] Whole wheat burger buns
- [ ] Lettuce, tomato, onion (for burger toppings)
- [ ] Salad greens (e.g., mixed greens, spinach)
- [ ] Salad dressin' of choice

Directions:

1. Mash black beans in a bowl until mostly smooth.
2. Form bean mixture into patties an' cook on a skillet or grill until heated through.
3. Toast whole wheat burger buns.
4. Assemble burgers with bean patties, lettuce, tomato, an' onion.
5. Serve with a side salad dressed with your favorite dressin'.

Nutrition Info per Servin' (approximately):

- Calories: 350
- Protein: 15g
- Fat: 8g
- Carbohydrates: 55g

Storage an' Freezin':

- Leftover bean patties can be refrigerated for up to 3 days or frozen for longer storage.

Why This Recipe is So Good:

- These black bean burgers are a nutritious alternative to traditional beef burgers, offerin' plant based protein an' plenty of fiber, served alongside a fresh an' crisp side salad.

Open Faced Turkey an' Avocado Sandwich on Whole Wheat Toast

Preparation Time: 10 minutes

Ingredients:

- [ ] Sliced turkey breast
- [ ] Avocado
- [ ] Whole wheat bread
- [ ] Lettuce
- [ ] Tomato

Directions:

1. Toast whole wheat bread slices until golden brown.
2. Mash avocado an' spread onto toast.
3. Layer sliced turkey, lettuce, an' tomato on top.
4. Serve open faced.

Nutrition Info per Servin' (approximately):

- Calories: 300
- Protein: 20g
- Fat: 10g
- Carbohydrates: 25g

Storage an' Freezin':

- Best enjoyed fresh.

Why This Recipe is So Good:

- This open faced sandwich is a delicious an' satisfyin' option, providin' lean protein from turkey an' healthy fats from avocado, all atop hearty whole wheat toast.

Gazpacho (Chilled Vegetable Soup)

Preparation Time: 15 minutes

Ingredients:

- [ ] Tomatoes
- [ ] Cucumber
- [ ] Bell peppers
- [ ] Onion
- [ ] Garlic
- [ ] Olive oil
- [ ] Vinegar
- [ ] Salt
- [ ] Pepper

Directions:

1. Blend tomatoes, cucumber, bell peppers, onion, an' garlic until smooth.
2. Stir in olive oil, vinegar, salt, an' pepper to taste.
3. Chill in the refrigerator for at least 1 hour before servin'.

Nutrition Info per Servin' (approximately):

- Calories: 120
- Protein: 2g
- Fat: 7g
- Carbohydrates: 15g

Storage an' Freezin':

- Gazpacho can be stored in the refrigerator for up to 3 days.

Why This Recipe is So Good:
- Gazpacho is a refreshin' an' hydratin' dish, loaded with vitamins an' minerals from fresh vegetables, perfect for a light an' nutritious meal option.

Chicken Caesar Salad (Use Light Caesar Dressin')

Preparation Time: 20 minutes

Ingredients:

- Grilled chicken breast
- Romaine lettuce
- Parmesan cheese
- Croutons
- Light Caesar dressin'

Directions:

1. Slice grilled chicken breast.
2. Toss romaine lettuce with grilled chicken, grated Parmesan cheese, croutons, an' light Caesar dressin'.
3. Serve immediately.

Nutrition Info per Servin' (approximately):

- Calories: 250
- Protein: 25g
- Fat: 10g
- Carbohydrates: 15g

Storage an' Freezin':

- Best enjoyed fresh.

Why This Recipe is So Good:

- This chicken Caesar salad offers a satisfyin' combination of protein rich chicken, crisp romaine lettuce, an' tangy Caesar dressin', makin' it a classic an' flavorful choice for a light meal.

Cobb Salad with Grilled Chicken or Fish

Preparation Time: 25 minutes

Ingredients:

- [ ] Grilled chicken or fish
- [ ] Salad greens (e.g., mixed greens, spinach)
- [ ] Hard boiled eggs
- [ ] Avocado
- [ ] Bacon (optional)
- [ ] Cherry tomatoes
- [ ] Blue cheese
- [ ] Salad dressin' of choice (e.g., vinaigrette)

Directions:

1. Chop grilled chicken or fish into bite sized pieces.
2. Arrange salad greens on a plate an' top with sliced hard boiled eggs, diced avocado, crumbled bacon (if usin'), halved cherry tomatoes, an' blue cheese.
3. Drizzle with salad dressin' of choice.
4. Serve immediately.

Nutrition Info per Servin' (approximately):

- Calories: 350
- Protein: 25g
- Fat: 20g
- Carbohydrates: 15g

Storage an' Freezin':

- Best enjoyed fresh.

Why This Recipe is So Good:
- Cobb salad is a hearty an' satisfyin' meal, loaded with protein, healthy fats, an' a variety of colorful vegetables, perfect for a nutritious an' flavorful lunch or dinner option.

Tuna Salad Sandwich on Whole Wheat Bread with Lettuce an' Tomato

Preparation Time: 10 minutes

Ingredients:

- [ ] Canned tuna
- [ ] Whole wheat bread
- [ ] Lettuce
- [ ] Tomato
- [ ] Mayonnaise or Greek yogurt (optional)

Directions:

1. Drain canned tuna an' place in a bowl.
2. Add mayonnaise or Greek yogurt if desired, then mix until combined.
3. Spread tuna salad onto whole wheat bread slices.
4. Top with lettuce an' tomato slices.
5. Cover with another slice of bread to make a sandwich.

Nutrition Info per Servin' (approximately):

- Calories: 250
- Protein: 20g
- Fat: 8g
- Carbohydrates: 25g

Storage an' Freezin':

- Best enjoyed fresh.

Why This Recipe is So Good:

- This tuna salad sandwich is a classic an' satisfyin' option, providin' a good source of protein an' fiber from the tuna an' whole wheat bread, perfect for a quick an' easy meal.

Turkey an' Swiss Roll Ups with Whole Wheat Tortillas an' Mustard

Preparation Time: 10 minutes

Ingredients:

- [ ] Sliced turkey breast
- [ ] Swiss cheese slices
- [ ] Whole wheat tortillas
- [ ] Mustard

Directions:

1. Lay out whole wheat tortillas on a flat surface.
2. Spread a thin layer of mustard over each tortilla.
3. Layer sliced turkey an' Swiss cheese on top of the tortillas.
4. Roll up tightly an' slice into pinwheels.

Nutrition Info per Servin' (approximately):

- Calories: 200
- Protein: 15g
- Fat: 8g
- Carbohydrates: 20g

Storage an' Freezin':

- Best enjoyed fresh.

Why This Recipe is So Good:

- These turkey an' Swiss roll ups are a convenient an' portable meal option, providin' protein an' whole grains, perfect for a quick an' satisfyin' lunch or snack.

Dinner

Baked Salmon with a Herb Crust an' Roasted Brussels Sprouts

Preparation Time: 25 minutes

Ingredients:

- [ ] Salmon fillets
- [ ] Fresh herbs (e.g., parsley, thyme, dill)
- [ ] Bread crumbs
- [ ] Olive oil
- [ ] Brussels sprouts

Directions:

1. Preheat oven to 400°F (200°C).
2. Mix chopped herbs with bread crumbs an' a drizzle of olive oil.
3. Press herb mixture onto the top of salmon fillets.
4. Place salmon on a bakin' sheet lined with parchment paper.
5. Toss Brussels sprouts with olive oil, salt, an' pepper, an' spread on the bakin' sheet around the salmon.
6. Bake for 15 20 minutes until salmon is cooked through an' Brussels sprouts are tender.

Nutrition Info per Servin' (approximately):

- Calories: 300
- Protein: 25g
- Fat: 15g
- Carbohydrates: 15g

Storage an' Freezin':

- Best enjoyed fresh.

Why This Recipe is So Good:

- It's a flavorful an' nutritious meal featurin' omega 3 rich salmon with a crispy herb crust, paired with roasted Brussels sprouts for a satisfyin' an' wholesome dinner.

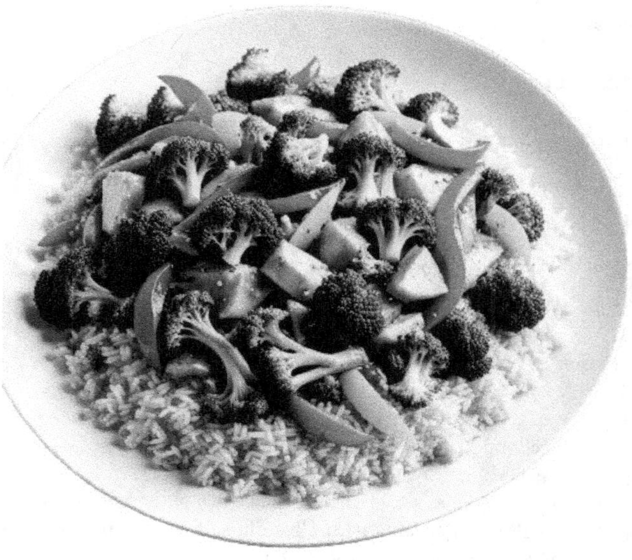

Chicken Stir Fry with Broccoli, Peppers, an' Brown Rice

Preparation Time: 30 minutes

Ingredients:

- ☐ Chicken breast, sliced
- ☐ Broccoli florets
- ☐ Bell peppers, sliced
- ☐ Brown rice
- ☐ Soy sauce
- ☐ Garlic
- ☐ Ginger
- ☐ Sesame oil

Directions:

1. Cook brown rice accordin' to package instructions.
2. Heat sesame oil in a large skillet or wok over medium high heat.
3. Add sliced chicken an' cook until browned.
4. Stir in minced garlic an' Ginger.
5. Add broccoli florets an' sliced bell peppers, cook until tender crisp.
6. Pour in soy sauce an' toss everythin' together.
7. Serve over cooked brown rice.

Nutrition Info per Servin' (approximately):

- Calories: 350
- Protein: 30g
- Fat: 10g
- Carbohydrates: 35g

Storage an' Freezin':
- Best enjoyed fresh.

Why This Recipe is So Good:
- It's a colorful an' flavorful stir fry packed with lean protein, crunchy veggies, an' whole grains, makin' it a balanced an' satisfyin' meal.

Turkey Meatloaf with Mashed Cauliflower (Use Low Fat Cheese)

Preparation Time: 1 hour

Ingredients:

- ☐ Ground turkey
- ☐ Bread crumbs
- ☐ Onion
- ☐ Garlic
- ☐ Egg
- ☐ Low fat cheese
- ☐ Cauliflower

Directions:

1. Preheat oven to 375°F (190°C).
2. Mix ground turkey with bread crumbs, chopped onion, minced garlic, beaten egg, an' shredded low fat cheese.
3. Form mixture into a loaf shape an' place in a bakin' dish.
4. Bake for 45 50 minutes until cooked through.
5. Meanwhile, steam cauliflower until tender, then mash until smooth.
6. Serve slices of turkey meatloaf with mashed cauliflower.

Nutrition Info per Servin' (approximately):

- Calories: 250
- Protein: 25g
- Fat: 10g
- Carbohydrates: 15g

Storage an' Freezin':

- Leftover meatloaf can be refrigerated for a few days. Mashed cauliflower is best enjoyed fresh.

Why This Recipe is So Good:

- It's a healthier twist on a classic comfort food, featurin' lean ground turkey an' creamy mashed cauliflower for a satisfyin' an' nutritious meal.

Shrimp Scampi over Whole Wheat Pasta (Use Sugar Free Marinara)

Preparation Time: 20 minutes

Ingredients:

- ☐ Shrimp
- ☐ Whole wheat pasta
- ☐ Garlic
- ☐ Lemon
- ☐ Olive oil
- ☐ Parsley
- ☐ Sugar free marinara sauce

Directions:

1. Cook whole wheat pasta accordin' to package instructions.
2. Heat olive oil in a skillet over medium heat, add minced garlic an' cook until fragrant.
3. Add shrimp to the skillet an' cook until pink an' opaque.
4. Squeeze fresh lemon juice over the shrimp.
5. Toss cooked pasta with sugar free marinara sauce.
6. Serve shrimp over pasta, garnished with chopped parsley.

Nutrition Info per Servin' (approximately):

- Calories: 300
- Protein: 25g
- Fat: 10g
- Carbohydrates: 30g

Storage an' Freezin':
- Best enjoyed fresh.

Why This Recipe is So Good:
- It's a light an' flavorful dish featurin' succulent shrimp cooked in garlic an' lemon, served over whole wheat pasta with a sugar free marinara sauce for a healthier twist on a classic favorite.

Lentil Bolognese with Zucchini Noodles

Preparation Time: 40 minutes

Ingredients:

- [ ] Lentils
- [ ] Zucchini
- [ ] Onion
- [ ] Garlic
- [ ] Tomato sauce
- [ ] Italian seasonin'

Directions:

1. Cook lentils accordin' to package instructions.
2. Spiralize zucchini into noodles.
3. In a skillet, sauté diced onion an' minced garlic until softened.
4. Add cooked lentils, tomato sauce, an' Italian seasonin' to the skillet, simmer for 10 minutes.
5. Sauté the zucchini noodles in a separate skillet until tender.
6. Serve lentil Bolognese over zucchini noodles.

Nutrition Info per Servin' (approximately):

- Calories: 250
- Protein: 15g
- Fat: 5g
- Carbohydrates: 40g

Storage an' Freezin':

- Leftover lentil Bolognese can be refrigerated for a few days. Zucchini noodles are best enjoyed fresh.

Why This Recipe is So Good:

- It's a hearty an' wholesome vegetarian alternative to traditional Bolognese, featurin' protein rich lentils an' low carb zucchini noodles for a nutritious an' satisfyin' meal.

Poached Chicken Breast with Quinoa an' Steamed Vegetables

Preparation Time: 30 minutes

Ingredients:

- ☐ Chicken breast
- ☐ Quinoa
- ☐ Assorted vegetables (e.g., broccoli, carrots, bell peppers)

Directions:

1. Season chicken breast with salt an' pepper.
2. Brin' a pot of water to a gentle simmer an' add the chicken breast.
3. Poach the chicken for about 15 20 minutes until cooked through.
4. Meanwhile, cook quinoa accordin' to package instructions.
5. Steam assorted vegetables until tender crisp.
6. Slice the poached chicken breast.
7. Serve sliced chicken over cooked quinoa with steamed vegetables on the side.

Nutrition Info per Servin' (approximately):

- Calories: 350
- Protein: 30g
- Fat: 5g
- Carbohydrates: 40g

Storage an' Freezin':

- Best enjoyed fresh.

Why This Recipe is So Good:

- It's a lean an' protein packed meal featurin' tender poached chicken breast, fiber rich quinoa, an' a variety of colorful steamed vegetables for a nutritious an' balanced dinner option.

Baked Tilapia with Lemon an' Dill Sauce, served with Roasted Sweet Potato

Preparation Time: 30 minutes

Ingredients:

- [ ] Tilapia fillets
- [ ] Lemon
- [ ] Fresh dill
- [ ] Greek yogurt
- [ ] Sweet potatoes

Directions:

1. Preheat oven to 375°F (190°C).
2. Season tilapia fillets with salt, pepper, an' lemon juice.
3. Place tilapia fillets on a bakin' sheet lined with parchment paper.
4. Bake for 15 20 minutes until fish is cooked through.
5. Meanwhile, mix Greek yogurt with chopped fresh dill an' a squeeze of lemon juice to make the sauce.
6. Roast sweet potatoes until tender.
7. Serve baked tilapia with lemon an' dill sauce, accompanied by roasted sweet potatoes.

Nutrition Info per Servin' (approximately):

- Calories: 250
- Protein: 25g
- Fat: 5g
- Carbohydrates: 30g

Storage an' Freezin':
- Best enjoyed fresh.

Why This Recipe is So Good:
- It's a light an' flavorful dish featurin' tender baked tilapia topped with a zesty lemon an' dill sauce, served alongside roasted sweet potatoes for a delicious an' nutritious meal option.

<u>Vegetarian Chili with Kidney Beans, Black Beans, an' Corn</u>

Preparation Time: 45 minutes

Ingredients:

- ☐ Kidney beans
- ☐ Black beans
- ☐ Corn kernels
- ☐ Onion
- ☐ Bell peppers
- ☐ Garlic
- ☐ Chili powder
- ☐ Cumin
- ☐ Crushed tomatoes

Directions:

1. In a large saucepan, warm olive oil over medium heat.
2. Sauté diced onion, minced garlic, an' chopped bell peppers until softened.
3. Add chili powder an' cumin, cook for a minute until fragrant.
4. Stir in drained kidney beans, black beans, corn kernels, an' crushed tomatoes.
5. Simmer for 30 minutes, stirrin' occasionally.
6. Adjust seasonin' with salt an' pepper to taste.
7. Serve hot, garnished with chopped cilantro an' a dollop of plain Greek yogurt if desired.

Nutrition Info per Servin' (approximately):

- Calories: 300
- Protein: 15g
- Fat: 5g
- Carbohydrates: 50g

Storage an' Freezin':

- Vegetarian chili can be refrigerated for up to 5 days or frozen for longer storage.

Why This Recipe is So Good:

- It's a hearty an' flavorful chili packed with protein an' fiber from kidney beans, black beans, an' corn, makin' it a satisfyin' an' comfortin' meal for vegetarians an' meat lovers alike.

Chicken Fajitas with Low Carb Tortillas, Grilled Peppers, an' Onions

Preparation Time: 25 minutes

Ingredients:

- ☐ Chicken breast
- ☐ Bell peppers
- ☐ Onion
- ☐ Fajita seasonin'
- ☐ Low carb tortillas

Directions:

1. Slice chicken breast into strips an' toss with fajita seasonin'.
2. Heat a grill pan or skillet over medium high heat.
3. Grill chicken until cooked through an' slightly charred.
4. Meanwhile, slice bell peppers an' onions into strips.
5. In the same pan, grill peppers an' onions until tender crisp.
6. Warm low carb tortillas on the grill for a few seconds on each side.
7. Serve grilled chicken, peppers, an' onions in low carb tortillas.

Nutrition Info per Servin' (approximately):

- Calories: 300
- Protein: 25g
- Fat: 10g
- Carbohydrates: 25g

Storage an' Freezin':

- Best enjoyed fresh.

Why This Recipe is So Good:

- It's a delicious an' satisfyin' Tex Mex favorite featurin' tender grilled chicken, sweet bell peppers, an' onions wrapped in low carb tortillas for a lighter yet flavorful meal option.

Turkey Burgers on Whole Wheat Buns with Sweet Potato Fries

Preparation Time: 40 minutes

Ingredients:

- ☐ Ground turkey
- ☐ Whole wheat burger buns
- ☐ Sweet potatoes
- ☐ Olive oil
- ☐ Seasonings (e.g., paprika, garlic powder)

Directions:

1. Preheat oven to 425°F (220°C).
2. Peel an' cut sweet potatoes into fries.
3. Toss sweet potato fries with olive oil an' seasonings.
4. Spread fries in a single layer on a bakin' sheet an' bake for 25 30 minutes, flippin' halfway through, until crispy.
5. Meanwhile, shape ground turkey into burger patties an' season with salt an' pepper.
6. Grill or cook turkey burgers in a skillet until cooked through.
7. Toast whole wheat burger buns.
8. Assemble burgers with turkey patties on buns an' serve with sweet potato fries.

Nutrition Info per Servin' (approximately):

- Calories: 400
- Protein: 25g
- Fat: 10g
- Carbohydrates: 50g

Storage an' Freezin':

- Leftover turkey burgers can be refrigerated for a few days. Sweet potato fries are best enjoyed fresh.

Why This Recipe is So Good:

- It's a healthier twist on a classic burger an' fries combo, featurin' lean turkey burgers on whole wheat buns paired with crispy sweet potato fries for a delicious an' satisfyin' meal option.

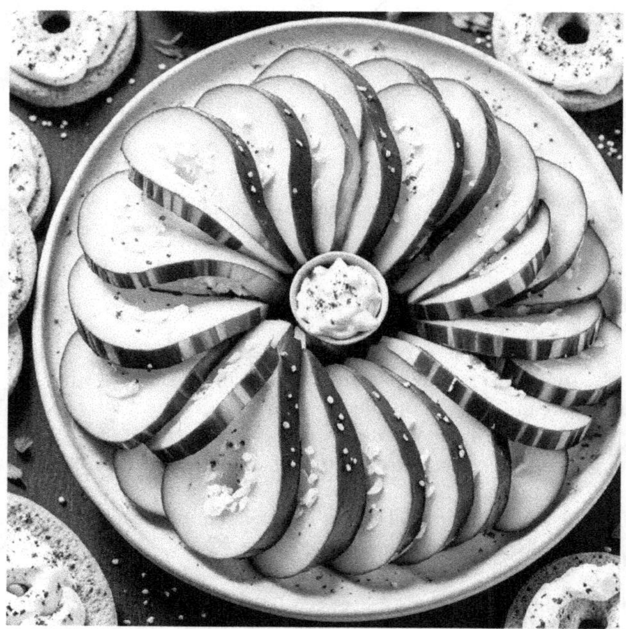

One Pan Chicken with Roasted Vegetables (Chicken Breasts, Broccoli, Carrots)

Preparation Time: 40 minutes

Ingredients:

- ☐ Chicken breasts
- ☐ Broccoli florets
- ☐ Carrots
- ☐ Olive oil
- ☐ Garlic powder
- ☐ Italian seasonin'

Directions:

1. Preheat oven to 425°F (220°C).
2. Arrange chicken breasts on one side of a bakin' sheet.
3. Toss broccoli florets an' sliced carrots with olive oil, garlic powder, an' Italian seasonin' on the other side of the bakin' sheet.
4. Season chicken breasts with salt an' pepper.
5. Roast everythin' in the oven for 25 30 minutes until chicken is cooked through an' vegetables are tender.
6. Serve chicken with roasted vegetables.

Nutrition Info per Servin' (approximately):

- Calories: 350
- Protein: 30g
- Fat: 10g
- Carbohydrates: 30g

Storage an' Freezin':

- Best enjoyed fresh.

Why This Recipe is So Good:

- It's a simple an' wholesome meal featurin' juicy chicken breasts roasted alongside flavorful broccoli an' carrots, all cooked on one pan for easy cleanup an' maximum flavor.

Baked Cod with Lemon an' Capers, served with Mashed Cauliflower

Preparation Time: 25 minutes

Ingredients:

- [ ] Cod fillets
- [ ] Lemon
- [ ] Capers
- [ ] Olive oil
- [ ] Garlic
- [ ] Cauliflower

Directions:

1. Preheat oven to 400°F (200°C).
2. Place cod fillets on a bakin' dish lined with parchment paper.
3. Drizzle with olive oil, sprinkle minced garlic, an' top with capers.
4. Squeeze fresh lemon juice over the fish.
5. Bake for 15 20 minutes until fish is opaque an' flakes easily with a fork.
6. Meanwhile, steam cauliflower until tender.
7. Mash cauliflower until smooth an' season with salt an' pepper.
8. Serve baked cod with mashed cauliflower on the side.

Nutrition Info per Servin' (approximately):

- Calories: 250
- Protein: 30g
- Fat: 10g
- Carbohydrates: 10g

Storage an' Freezin':

- Best enjoyed fresh.

Why This Recipe is So Good:

- It's a light an' flavorful dish featurin' tender baked cod with a zesty lemon an' caper toppin', served alongside creamy mashed cauliflower for a satisfyin' an' nutritious meal option.

Stuffed Peppers with Ground Turkey, Brown Rice, an' Vegetables

Preparation Time: 50 minutes

Ingredients:

- [ ] Bell peppers
- [ ] Ground turkey
- [ ] Brown rice
- [ ] Onion
- [ ] Garlic
- [ ] Tomato sauce

Directions:

1. Preheat oven to 375°F (190°C).
2. Cut the tops off bell peppers an' remove seeds an' membranes.
3. Cook brown rice accordin' to package instructions.
4. In a skillet, cook ground turkey with diced onion an' minced garlic until browned.
5. Stir in cooked brown rice an' tomato sauce, cook for a few more minutes.
6. Spoon turkey an' rice mixture into bell peppers.
7. Place stuffed peppers in a bakin' dish, cover with foil, an' bake for 30 - 35 minutes until peppers are tender.

Nutrition Info per Servin' (approximately):

- Calories: 300
- Protein: 20g
- Fat: 10g
- Carbohydrates: 30g

Storage an' Freezin':

- Stuffed peppers can be refrigerated for a few days or frozen for longer storage.

Why This Recipe is So Good:

- It's a wholesome an' satisfyin' meal featurin' tender bell peppers stuffed with a flavorful mixture of lean ground turkey, nutty brown rice, an' savory vegetables, makin' it a delicious an' nutritious option for lunch or dinner.

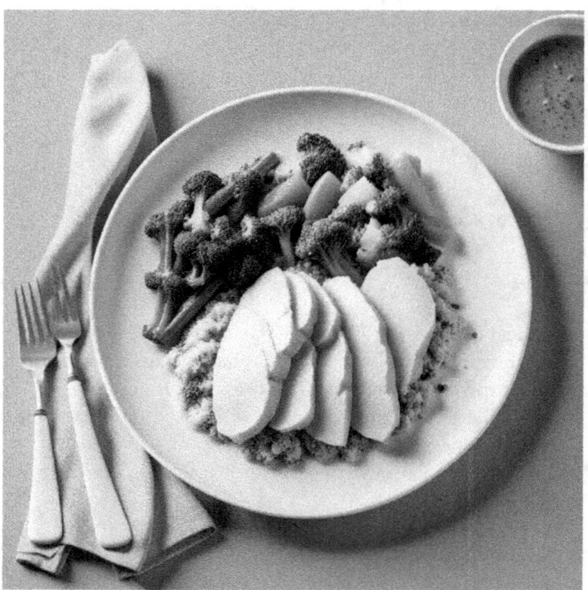

Chicken an' Vegetable Curry with Cauliflower Rice

Preparation Time: 40 minutes

Ingredients:

- ☐ Chicken thighs
- ☐ Assorted vegetables (e.g., bell peppers, carrots, peas)
- ☐ Curry paste
- ☐ Coconut milk
- ☐ Cauliflower

Directions:

1. Cut chicken thighs into bite sized pieces.
2. In a large skillet, cook chicken until browned.
3. Add diced vegetables an' cook until softened.
4. Stir in curry paste an' coconut milk, simmer for 15 20 minutes.
5. Meanwhile, pulse cauliflower in a food processor to make cauliflower rice.
6. Heat cauliflower rice in a separate skillet until tender.
7. Serve chicken an' vegetable curry over cauliflower rice.

Nutrition Info per Servin' (approximately):

- Calories: 350
- Protein: 25g
- Fat: 15g
- Carbohydrates: 20g

Storage an' Freezin':

- Best enjoyed fresh.

Why This Recipe is So Good:

- It's a fragrant an' flavorful curry featurin' tender chicken an' colorful vegetables in a creamy coconut sauce, served over low carb cauliflower rice for a lighter yet satisfyin' meal option.

Vegetarian Chili with a Dollop of Plain Greek Yogurt

Preparation Time: 45 minutes

Ingredients:

- ☐ Kidney beans
- ☐ Black beans
- ☐ Corn kernels
- ☐ Onion
- ☐ Bell peppers
- ☐ Garlic
- ☐ Chili powder
- ☐ Cumin
- ☐ Crushed tomatoes
- ☐ Plain Greek yogurt

Directions:

1. In a large saucepan, warm olive oil over medium heat.
2. Sauté diced onion, minced garlic, an' chopped bell peppers until softened.
3. Add chili powder an' cumin, cook for a minute until fragrant.
4. Stir in drained kidney beans, black beans, corn kernels, an' crushed tomatoes.
5. Simmer for 30 minutes, stirrin' occasionally.
6. Adjust seasonin' with salt an' pepper to taste.
7. Serve hot, garnished with a dollop of plain Greek yogurt.

Nutrition Info per Servin' (approximately):

- Calories: 300
- Protein: 15g
- Fat: 5g
- Carbohydrates: 50g

Storage an' Freezin':

- Vegetarian chili can be refrigerated for up to 5 days or frozen for longer storage.

Why This Recipe is So Good:

- It's a hearty an' flavorful chili packed with protein an' fiber from kidney beans, black beans, an' corn, an' topped with creamy Greek yogurt for a delicious an' nutritious meal option.

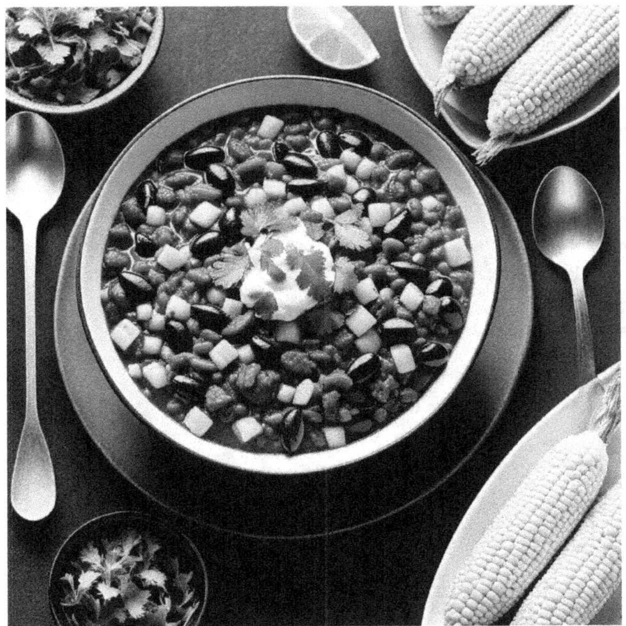

Snacks

Celery Sticks with Almond Butter

Preparation Time: 5 minutes

Ingredients:

- [ ] Celery sticks
- [ ] Almond butter

Directions:

1. Wash an' trim celery sticks.
2. Fill the celery with almond butter.
3. Serve immediately.

Nutrition Info per Servin' (approximately):

- Calories: 100
- Protein: 3g
- Fat: 8g
- Carbohydrates: 4g

Storage an' Freezin':

- Best enjoyed fresh.

Why This Snack is So Good:

- It's a crunchy, satisfyin' snack rich in fiber, healthy fats, an' protein, makin' it a perfect pick me up.

Handful of Almonds an' Dried Cranberries

Preparation Time: Instant

Ingredients:

- [ ] Almonds
- [ ] Dried cranberries

Directions:

1. Simply combine almonds an' dried cranberries in a bowl.
2. Enjoy as is.

Nutrition Info per Servin' (approximately):

- Calories: 150
- Protein: 5g
- Fat: 10g
- Carbohydrates: 14g

Storage an' Freezin':

- Store in an airtight container for a grab an' go snack.

Why This Snack is So Good:

- It offers a satisfyin' mix of protein, healthy fats, an' a touch of sweetness from the cranberries, perfect for an energy boost between meals.

Cottage Cheese with Sliced Cucumber an' Tomato

Preparation Time: 5 minutes

Ingredients:

- [ ] Cottage cheese
- [ ] Cucumber
- [ ] Tomato

Directions:

1. Arrange cottage cheese on a plate.
2. Top with sliced cucumber an' tomato.
3. Serve immediately.

Nutrition Info per Servin' (approximately):

- Calories: 120
- Protein: 12g
- Fat: 3g
- Carbohydrates: 10g

Storage an' Freezin':

- Best enjoyed fresh.

Why This Snack is So Good:

- It's a light an' refreshin' snack packed with protein, vitamins, an' minerals, perfect for a quick an' healthy bite.

Hard Boiled Egg

Preparation Time: 10 minutes

Ingredients:

☐ Eggs

Directions:

1. Place eggs in a saucepan an' cover with water.
2. Brin' water to a boil, then reduce heat an' simmer for 10 12 minutes.
3. Remove eggs from water an' let cool before peelin'.
4. Serve whole or sliced.

Nutrition Info per Servin' (approximately):

- Calories: 70
- Protein: 6g
- Fat: 5g
- Carbohydrates: 0g

Storage an' Freezin':

- Hard boiled eggs can be stored in the refrigerator for up to one week.

Why This Snack is So Good:

- Eggs are a nutrient powerhouse, providin' high quality protein an' essential vitamins an' minerals, makin' them a convenient an' satisfyin' snack.

Sliced Bell Peppers with Hummus

Preparation Time: 5 minutes

Ingredients:

- ☐ Bell peppers (various colors)
- ☐ Hummus

Directions:

1. Wash an' slice bell peppers into strips.
2. Serve with hummus for dippin'.

Nutrition Info per Servin' (approximately):

- Calories: 80
- Protein: 3g
- Fat: 4g
- Carbohydrates: 10g

Storage an' Freezin':

- Best enjoyed fresh.

Why This Snack is So Good:

- It's a colorful an' crunchy snack loaded with vitamins, fiber, an' healthy fats from the hummus, perfect for satisfyin' hunger an' boostin' energy.

Greek Yogurt with a Sprinkle of Cinnamon an' Chopped Walnuts

Preparation Time: Instant

Ingredients:

- ☐ Greek yogurt
- ☐ Cinnamon
- ☐ Walnuts

Directions:

- Spoon Greek yogurt into a bowl.
- Sprinkle with cinnamon an' chopped walnuts.
- Serve immediately.

Nutrition Info per Servin' (approximately):

- Calories: 150
- Protein: 15g
- Fat: 7g
- Carbohydrates: 8g

Storage an' Freezin':

- Best enjoyed fresh.

Why This Snack is So Good:

- Greek yogurt provides protein an' probiotics while cinnamon adds flavor an' walnuts offer crunch an' healthy fats, creatin' a delicious an' nutritious snack option.

Sugar Free Applesauce

Preparation Time: Instant

Ingredients:

- [ ] Applesauce (sugar free)

Directions:

1. Simply open the container of sugar free applesauce.
2. Serve chilled or at room temperature.

Nutrition Info per Servin' (approximately):

- Calories: 50
- Protein: 0g
- Fat: 0g
- Carbohydrates: 12g

Storage an' Freezin':

- Store in the refrigerator after openin'.

Why This Snack is So Good:

- It's a low calorie, naturally sweet snack option packed with fiber an' vitamins from apples, perfect for satisfyin' cravings without added sugars.

Cucumber Slices with Low Fat Cream Cheese an' Everythin' Bagel Seasonin'

Preparation Time: 5 minutes

Ingredients:

- ☐ Cucumber
- ☐ Low fat cream cheese
- ☐ Everythin' bagel seasonin'

Directions:

1. Slice cucumber into rounds.
2. Spread low fat cream cheese on each slice.
3. Sprinkle with everythin' bagel seasonin'.

Nutrition Info per Servin' (approximately):

Calories: 60
Protein: 2g
Fat: 3g
Carbohydrates: 5g

Storage an' Freezin':

- Best enjoyed fresh.

Why This Snack is So Good:

- It's a light an' flavorful snack packed with hydratin' cucumber, protein rich cream cheese, an' savory seasonin', offerin' a satisfyin' crunch an' taste.

Edamame Pods

Preparation Time: 5 minutes

Ingredients:

- [ ] Edamame pods (frozen or fresh)
- [ ] Salt (optional)

Directions:

1. Boil or steam edamame pods accordin' to package instructions.
2. Drain an' season with salt if desired.
3. Serve warm or chilled.

Nutrition Info per Servin' (approximately):

- Calories: 100
- Protein: 8g
- Fat: 3g
- Carbohydrates: 9g

Storage an' Freezin':

- Store in the refrigerator if cooked, or freeze if raw.

Why This Snack is So Good:

- Edamame pods are a protein packed snack rich in fiber, vitamins, an' minerals, offerin' a satisfyingly crunchy texture an' delicious flavor.

Air Popped Popcorn with a Sprinkle of Parmesan Cheese

Preparation Time: 5 minutes

Ingredients:

- [ ] Popcorn kernels
- [ ] Parmesan cheese (grated)

Directions:

1. Air pop popcorn usin' a popcorn maker or stovetop method.
2. Sprinkle with grated Parmesan cheese while still warm.
3. Toss to coat evenly an' serve immediately.

Nutrition Info per Servin' (approximately):

- Calories: 80
- Protein: 3g
- Fat: 3g
- Carbohydrates: 12g

Storage an' Freezin':

- Best enjoyed fresh.

Why This Snack is So Good:

- It's a satisfyin' an' savory snack low in calories an' high in fiber, offerin' a guilt free indulgence with a boost of cheesy flavor.

Week 1 Meal Plan

Day 1:

- [ ] Breakfast: Chia Seed Puddin' with Nut Butter an' Sliced Strawberries
- [ ] Lunch: Chicken or Turkey Lettuce Wraps with chopped vegetables an' a low sugar peanut sauce
- [ ] Dinner: Baked Salmon with a herb crust an' roasted Brussels sprouts
- [ ] Snacks (choose 2): Celery sticks with almond butter, Handful of almonds an' dried cranberries

Day 2:

- [ ] Breakfast: Scrambled Eggs with Spinach an' Feta Cheese
- [ ] Lunch: Lentil Soup with whole wheat bread for dippin'
- [ ] Dinner: Chicken Stir Fry with broccoli, peppers, an' brown rice
- [ ] Snacks (choose 2): Cottage cheese with sliced cucumber an' tomato, Hard boiled egg

Day 3:

- [ ] Breakfast: Greek Yogurt with Chopped Nuts an' a sprinkle of berries
- [ ] Lunch: Grilled poultry or fish paired with roasted vegetables
- [ ] Dinner: Turkey Meatloaf with mashed cauliflower (use low fat cheese)
- [ ] Snacks (choose 2): Sliced bell peppers with hummus, Greek yogurt with a sprinkle of cinnamon an' chopped walnuts

Day 4:

- [ ] Breakfast: Protein Smoothie with Berries an' Unsweetened Almond Milk
- [ ] Lunch: Leftover stir fry from Day 2 (ensure low sugar ingredients)
- [ ] Dinner: Shrimp Scampi over whole wheat pasta (use sugar free marinara)
- [ ] Snacks (choose 2): Sugar free applesauce, Cucumber slices with low fat cream cheese an' everythin' bagel seasonin'

Day 5:

- [ ] Breakfast: Baked Oatmeal with Apples an' Cinnamon (use sugar substitutes like stevia)
- [ ] Lunch: Tuna Salad on a bed of romaine lettuce with chopped celery an' red onion
- [ ] Dinner: Lentil Bolognese with zucchini noodles
- [ ] Snacks (choose 2): Edamame pods, Air popped popcorn with a sprinkle of Parmesan cheese

Day 6:

- [ ] Breakfast: Poached Eggs on a bed of wilted greens
- [ ] Lunch: Black Bean Burgers on whole wheat buns with a side salad
- [ ] Dinner: Baked Tilapia with lemon an' dill sauce, served with roasted sweet potato
- [ ] Snacks (choose 2): Celery sticks with almond butter, Handful of almonds an' dried cranberries

Day 7:

- [ ] Breakfast: Whole Wheat Toast with Avocado an' a sprinkle of Everythin' But the Bagel Seasonin'
- [ ] Lunch: Chicken Caesar Salad (use light Caesar dressin')
- [ ] Dinner: Vegetarian Chili with kidney beans, black beans, an' corn (add a dollop of plain Greek yogurt if tolerated)
- [ ] Snacks (choose 2): Cottage cheese with sliced cucumber an' tomato, Hard boiled egg

Week 2 Meal Plan

Day 1:

- [ ] Breakfast: Cottage Cheese Pancakes with a dollop of sugar free syrup
- [ ] Lunch: Cold Sesame Noodles with shredded chicken an' vegetables (use low sugar sesame sauce)
- [ ] Dinner: Vegetarian Chili with kidney beans, black beans, an' corn
- [ ] Snacks (choose 2): Greek yogurt with a sprinkle of cinnamon an' chopped walnuts, Air popped popcorn with a sprinkle of Parmesan cheese

Day 2:

- [ ] Breakfast: Savory Frittata with Vegetables an' Goat Cheese
- [ ] Lunch: Tuna Salad Sandwich on whole wheat bread with lettuce an' tomato
- [ ] Dinner: Chicken Fajitas with low carb tortillas, grilled peppers an' onions
- [ ] Snacks (choose 2): Celery sticks with almond butter, Hard boiled egg

Day 3:

- [ ] Breakfast: Protein Smoothie with Berries an' Unsweetened Almond Milk
- [ ] Lunch: Gazpacho (chilled vegetable soup)
- [ ] Dinner: Baked Cod with lemon an' capers, served with mashed cauliflower
- [ ] Snacks (choose 2): Handful of almonds an' dried cranberries, Sliced bell peppers with hummus

Day 4:

- [ ] Breakfast: Whole Wheat Toast with Avocado an' a sprinkle of Everythin' But the Bagel Seasonin'
- [ ] Lunch: Turkey an' Swiss Roll Ups with whole wheat tortillas an' mustard
- [ ] Dinner: Poached Chicken Breast with quinoa an' steamed vegetables
- [ ] Snacks (choose 2): Cottage cheese with sliced cucumber an' tomato, Sugar free applesauce

Day 5:

- [ ] Breakfast: Scrambled Eggs with Spinach an' Feta Cheese
- [ ] Lunch: Black Bean Burgers on whole wheat buns with a side salad (omit dressin' or use light vinaigrette)
- [ ] Dinner: One Pan Chicken with roasted vegetables (chicken breasts, broccoli, carrots)
- [ ] Snacks (choose 2): Edamame pods, Greek yogurt with a sprinkle of cinnamon an' chopped walnuts

Day 6:

- [ ] Breakfast: Baked Oatmeal with Apples an' Cinnamon (use sugar substitutes like stevia)
- [ ] Lunch: Chicken Caesar Salad (use light Caesar dressin')
- [ ] Dinner: Stuffed Peppers with ground turkey, brown rice, an' vegetables
- [ ] Snacks (choose 2): Celery sticks with almond butter, Handful of almonds an' dried cranberries

Day 7:

- [ ] Breakfast: Greek Yogurt with Chopped Nuts an' a sprinkle of berries
- [ ] Lunch: Lentil Soup with whole wheat bread for dippin'
- [ ] Dinner: Shrimp Scampi over whole wheat pasta (use sugar free marinara)
- [ ] Snacks (choose 2): Cucumber slices with low fat cream cheese an' everythin' bagel seasonin', Air popped popcorn with a sprinkle of Parmesan cheese

Week 3 Meal Plan

Day 1:

- [ ] Breakfast: Protein Smoothie with Berries an' Unsweetened Almond Milk (add a scoop of protein powder for extra satiety)
- [ ] Lunch: Turkey an' Vegetable Chili (use no sugar added diced tomatoes) with a dollop of plain Greek yogurt
- [ ] Dinner: Baked Tilapia with lemon an' dill sauce, served with roasted sweet potato wedges (cut sweet potato into smaller pieces for easier digestion)
- [ ] Snacks (choose 2): Edamame pods, Cottage cheese with sliced cucumber an' tomato

Day 2:

- [ ] Breakfast: Poached Eggs on a bed of wilted greens with a drizzle of olive oil an' lemon juice
- [ ] Lunch: Chicken or Turkey Lettuce Wraps with chopped vegetables an' a low sugar peanut sauce (thin the sauce with a little water for easier consumption)
- [ ] Dinner: Vegetarian Chili with kidney beans, black beans, an' corn (puree a portion for a smoother consistency if needed)
- [ ] Snacks (choose 2): Handful of almonds an' dried cranberries, Celery sticks with almond butter

Day 3:

- [ ] Breakfast: Whole Wheat Toast with mashed avocado an' a sprinkle of Everythin' But the Bagel Seasonin'
- [ ] Lunch: Cobb Salad with grilled chicken or fish (opt for grilled fish for a lighter option)
- [ ] Dinner: Shrimp Scampi over whole wheat pasta (use sugar free marinara, cut pasta into smaller pieces)
- [ ] Snacks (choose 2): Greek yogurt with a sprinkle of cinnamon an' chopped walnuts, Sliced bell peppers with hummus

Day 4:

- [ ] Breakfast: Scrambled Eggs with Spinach an' Feta Cheese

- [ ] Lunch: Black Bean Burgers on whole wheat buns with a side salad (use a light vinaigrette dressin')
- [ ] Dinner: One Pan Chicken with roasted vegetables (chicken breasts, broccoli, carrots) (cut vegetables into bite sized pieces for easier digestion)
- [ ] Snacks (choose 2): Sugar free applesauce, Air popped popcorn with a sprinkle of Parmesan cheese

Day 5:

- [ ] Breakfast: Chia Seed Puddin' with Nut Butter an' Sliced Strawberries
- [ ] Lunch: Tuna Salad on a bed of romaine lettuce with chopped celery an' red onion
- [ ] Dinner: Lentil Bolognese with zucchini noodles (ensure lentils are well cooked for easier digestion)
- [ ] Snacks (choose 2): Hard boiled egg, Cucumber slices with low fat cream cheese an' everythin' bagel seasonin'

Day 6:

- [ ] Breakfast: Baked Oatmeal with Apples an' Cinnamon (use a minimal amount of sugar substitute)
- [ ] Lunch: Gazpacho (chilled vegetable soup) (ensure vegetables are blended smooth for easier consumption)
- [ ] Dinner: Stuffed Peppers with ground turkey, brown rice (opt for white rice if brown rice is too difficult to digest), an' vegetables
- [ ] Snacks (choose 2): Celery sticks with almond butter, Handful of almonds an' dried cranberries

Day 7:

- [ ] Breakfast: Greek Yogurt with Chopped Nuts an' a sprinkle of berries
- [ ] Lunch: Chicken Caesar Salad (use light Caesar dressin', opt for grilled chicken for a lighter option)
- [ ] Dinner: Salmon with a lemon dill sauce an' steamed asparagus
- [ ] Snacks (choose 2): Cottage cheese with sliced cucumber an' tomato, Edamame pods

Week 4 Meal Plan

Day 1:

- [ ] Breakfast: Smoothie with plain Greek yogurt, berries, an' unsweetened almond milk (blended smooth)
- [ ] Lunch: Cream of Wheat cereal cooked with unsweetened almond milk an' mashed banana (thin with additional milk if needed)
- [ ] Dinner: Salmon with lemon dill sauce, steamed an' puréed with a side of mashed sweet potato (use low fat milk or broth for mashin')
- [ ] Snacks (choose 2): Applesauce, Cottage cheese with mashed avocado

Day 2:

- [ ] Breakfast: Scrambled eggs with chopped spinach an' feta cheese, puréed after cookin'
- [ ] Lunch: Chicken or turkey soup with finely chopped vegetables (ensure vegetables are very soft)
- [ ] Dinner: Vegetarian chili with kidney beans, black beans, an' corn, puréed for a smoother consistency
- [ ] Snacks (choose 2): Mashed banana with a sprinkle of cinnamon, Yogurt with mashed berries

Day 3:

- [ ] Breakfast: Chia seed puddin' with nut butter an' mashed strawberries (ensure chia seeds are softened)
- [ ] Lunch: Tuna salad with mashed avocado on whole wheat toast (cut toast into bite sized pieces)
- [ ] Dinner: Baked cod with lemon an' capers, flaked an' served with mashed cauliflower
- [ ] Snacks (choose 2): Cottage cheese with mashed pear, Steamed an' mashed broccoli florets

Day 4:

- [ ] Breakfast: Protein smoothie with berries, unsweetened almond milk, an' a scoop of protein powder (blended smooth)

- [ ] Lunch: Lentil soup with well cooked lentils an' finely chopped vegetables, puréed for a smoother consistency
- [ ] Dinner: Chicken stir fry with broccoli, peppers, an' brown rice (ensure chicken is shredded an' vegetables are very soft)
- [ ] Snacks (choose 2): Mashed sweet potato with a sprinkle of cinnamon, Yogurt with mashed banana

Day 5:

- [ ] Breakfast: Scrambled eggs with chopped mushrooms an' a sprinkle of cheese, puréed after cookin'
- [ ] Lunch: Black bean burger on a whole wheat bun, mashed with a fork for easier consumption
- [ ] Dinner: One pan chicken with roasted vegetables (chicken breasts, broccoli, carrots) all ingredients puréed after cookin'
- [ ] Snacks (choose 2): Applesauce with a sprinkle of ground Ginger, Mashed avocado with a squeeze of lemon juice

Day 6:

- [ ] Breakfast: Oatmeal with mashed banana an' a sprinkle of cinnamon, cooked with unsweetened almond milk
- [ ] Lunch: Gazpacho (chilled vegetable soup) ensure all vegetables are blended very smooth
- [ ] Dinner: Turkey meatloaf with mashed cauliflower (use low fat cheese an' ensure meatloaf is well cooked an' soft)
- [ ] Snacks (choose 2): Cottage cheese with mashed berries, Steamed an' mashed green beans

Day 7:

- [ ] Breakfast: Greek yogurt with mashed berries an' a sprinkle of chopped nuts
- [ ] Lunch: Chicken Caesar salad with grilled chicken (cut chicken into bite sized pieces, opt for light Caesar dressin')
- [ ] Dinner: Shrimp scampi over whole wheat pasta (use sugar free marinara, cut pasta into small pieces, ensure shrimp are well cooked an' soft)
- [ ] Snacks (choose 2): Mashed avocado with a sprinkle of lemon juice, Yogurt with mashed banana an' a sprinkle of chia seeds

Thank you for Reading

www.ingramcontent.com/pod-product-compliance
Lightning Source LLC
Chambersburg PA
CBHW071224260726

48653CB00042B/2304